You Were Stabbed Where?

Real Stories from a Small-Town ER

Kerry Hamm

Edited for quality purposes after publication.

If you haven't read the first two books, don't worry. Let me fill you in on a few things:

Welcome to a small-town Emergency Room in Ohio. With six trauma bays, one mental health room, one low pressure room, one quarantine room, and 11 other exam bays, this ER has the capacity to fit 21 patients at a time, with more than 100 patients often lining up in the lobby and waiting room on any given evening shift.

We're no big-shot inner city hospital. We transfer out burns and severe pediatric cases. We have a mental health floor, inpatient rehab, intermediate care/critical care, and hospice floor in addition to pediatrics, general surgery, obstetrics, and nursery floors. Unless patients are directly admitted from facilities in surrounding areas, they show up in our department first.

In my other two books, I said we don't typically see a lot of stabbings or gunshot wounds.

This apparently jinxed us, because this book is filled with the first of the two.

My name is Kerry and I'm the first person you'll see when you come through those ER doors: registration. Two to three clerks work during the day and evening shifts, taking turns gathering names, birth dates, and diagnoses at the front (while juggling floor transfers, admits from surrounding hospitals, and outside phone calls from some cat lady named Linda who's making her third call this shift to see if we think she needs to come in for tingling in her left butt cheek), and then in the back, where we enter patients' rooms to gather contact and insurance information to complete the registration process.

It used to be, once 11 p.m. hit, I waved to my coworkers as they walked out the door, and I was left at the registration desk with a triage nurse in a small room behind the desk, security lurking behind a two-way mirror that takes up an entire wall in front of the registration desk, a not-so-empty waiting room to my right, and six registered nurses and one or two doctors in the back.

Well, it turns out someone was paying attention, so a few days out of my week-long stretches, I have an awesome coworker at my side for a couple of hours.

Every story here is true, though dialogue has been changed slightly, all names have been changed, and some situations have been slightly altered to protect patient privacy. It has never been my intention to exploit the heartaches or embarrassments of others, but simply offer a glimpse into the world of the Emergency Room, where every patient seems to be a wild card.

Crazy Isn't a Costume

Halloween night was fairly quiet at our hospital. Sure, we had the occasional patient in a costume, but nobody was dressed in outrageous garb. We saw a few Sock Hop girls in poodle skirts and saddle shoes, a 'zombie vampire,' and a handful of children still wearing Power Ranger and Minion costumes presenting with tummy aches and leg pain after walking for hours around the town and sneaking candy the whole way home.

A little after midnight, a man wearing a black hoodie and torn jeans entered the lobby. Something was 'off' about him. He seemed jittery and unfocused. His fingers trembled and his left eyebrow twitched. My first thought, honestly, was that he was on drugs. It would only make sense that someone like this would come in when all was quiet.

More obvious than the man's nervous behavior, though, was a Japanese sword in a sheath that stretched across his back and was tied to the center of his chest with a thin canvas strap.

"Can I help you?" I asked.

The man opened his mouth to speak, but nothing came out but a few incoherent stammers.

"Do you need to see a doctor?"

My coworker eyed the man.

I looked over to the security office and hoped

someone was in there to keep an extra watch.

The man approached the desk in a stagger and then something clicked from deep within. His stare became hard and dark; his hands became steady. He seemed more confident and there was a twinge of anger glimmering from his midnight eyes.

And then he reached for the sword.

One of our security guards flew out of their office and burst into the lobby before the man could remove the sword from the sheath.

"Sir," said the guard, "we can't allow weapons on the property."

The odd man seemed taken aback by this statement but didn't remove his hand from the sword's handle. Instead, he seemed to challenge the guard with a resentful glare.

"If you are here for medical attention," the guard continued, "I have to hold any weapons you may have until you are discharged."

We all watched the man. He dropped his arm and slouched his shoulders.

"It's a toy," he chuckled nervously. "It's part of my costume."

His declaration wasn't incredibly reassuring. I don't know about anyone else in the room, but I didn't believe the man.

"Well," the guard said, "if you don't mind handing it over for inspection..."

The man shook his head violently. "No. No.

I told you, it's just a toy. No. You can't touch it. You can't have it. Nobody can touch it."

"Then I'll have to ask you to leave the property," said the guard.

I thought the man would argue, but he didn't. Instead, he left the property while muttering words none of us caught.

The next night, the man came back again, dressed in the same outfit from before—sans sword. Instead, he carried a few grocery sacks filled with clothes and DVDs. He wanted to speak to a doctor regarding mental health.

For whatever reason, the patient was not admitted to the mental health floor after speaking to the ER doctor and mental health duty counselor. It's not uncommon to see patients discharged after speaking to professionals, and I usually don't think anything of it.

I thought something of it when the patient exited the ER and pulled a hunting knife from his pocket. And when I say knife, let's all think back to *Crocodile Dundee*. What this man removed from his pocket sure was a knife, and it was a big one. He poked at his palm with the sharp tip until blood dripped to the lobby floor.

Trying not to draw attention to myself, I moved slowly to pick up the phone and dial security. When they didn't answer, the call forwarded to the operator, and she informed me security was called to a disturbance on another floor. They would be unavailable for "at least a few minutes."

That, obviously, wasn't a great answer to hear. Almost in a whisper, I told the operator at least one security officer was needed in the ER lobby as soon as possible.

By the time security arrived, the discharged cut-happy patient was in the parking lot. A few nurses and I watched him on the security camera monitors to the left of the registration desk. He was wandering in large circles, going between waving the knife in the air and poking at his palm some more.

Security cautiously approached the patient and the mental health duty counselor was informed of the situation. The patient walked off hospital property in the middle of all of this and was later arrested for public intoxication.

Evasion

I'd just gotten to work and took a quick look at the Tracking Board. We weren't getting slammed or anything, but we weren't able to sit back and reflect on life or whatever people do when they're not busy. I'd give a better example, really, but when the staff on our shifts aren't busy, we're usually sighing in relief that it's all over and then scrambling to catch up on paperwork before the next rush blows through.

None of the patients on the board presented with anything life-threatening. Three of the patients had chief complaints of congestion. One child had a complaint of laceration to forehead. Half of the patients in the back were marked as discharged and were only waiting for discharge papers before they could leave.

As patients continued to come and go, I went to the back part of the office and worked on catching up on reports from the night before. I knew my coworker was about to leave and I would be alone on the overnight shift, so I was rushing through my work at the speed of light.

"I need help," I heard a man yell.

I hurried to the registration desk and saw a man holding his young daughter. Blood was smeared all over her cheeks and down her chin. I immediately recognized the patient and her father as frequent flyers.

"What happened?" I asked, as I handed the father a washrag.

He shrugged. "We were driving and looked back to see blood all over her. She was sleeping when it started."

I stopped. "Wait. Didn't I see you leave here about a twenty minutes ago?"

"Yeah," he nodded. He motioned to the girl. "She was throwing up earlier."

I registered the patient for her second visit that night and explained to the father that the only waiting time he would experience this time around would be the time it took for the triage nurse to walk from the back to front after I called her. He was okay with that. I called the nurse, printed the patient's labels, and started stickering her papers: two forms for the triage nurse to chart on, the patient's consent form, and her ID band.

Before I could finish stickering the papers, and just as the triage nurse entered the triage room, the patient's mother stomped inside and shouted as she made her way to the waiting room, "We're going to a different hospital. Now."

"Ma'am," I said, "your daughter is ready to be seen right now. There's not a wait, if that's what you're worried about."

"It's not," she sneered. She ordered her husband, "Let's go. We're leaving."

As the father carried the patient outside, the

family passed a cop coming inside. The officer came to the desk and put his palms down.

"So?" he asked.

I shrugged. "So?"

"Did those people get here okay?"

"No idea what you're talking about," I laughed.

"Oh, I guess it wasn't you I was talking to. I guess a woman called 911 and said they were avoiding a unit because they were on the way here with a bleeding child."

I pointed to the parking lot. "I'm pretty sure you passed them on the way in."

He whipped his head around and watched the family's car pull away. "You mean they left? Did they even check in?"

I nodded and explained what happened. The officer radioed another nearby unit and the family was pulled over for a missing taillight, as well as a wellness check stemming from the 911 call.

That wasn't all the family received. Mom admitted dad was speeding and she had the 'bright idea' to call 911 to escape a ticket. Nobody explained to us how the child became bloodied, but we used our imaginations.

Update: I figured I'd add an update while I was cleaning up some missed mistakes. After an investigation, authorities found the child was abused in order for the parents to avoid a ticket.

Their children were removed from their custody for the time being, and the parents have both presented to the ER since then.

I keep seeing the word 'chronic' in diagnoses and charts.

Chronic back pain. Chronic kidney pain. Chronic leg pain.

Can we all, PLEASE, vote in the usage of 'chronic poor life choices?'

Hard Not to Draw Conclusions

A call came over the ambulance scanner at two in the morning. EMS were en route to a six-year-old boy experiencing a choking episode. We expected the ambulance to arrive shortly, and we figured we'd have a few hysterical family members at the front desk.

While the ambulance did arrive shortly after the call came through, the lobby wasn't flooded with family members. In fact, I ran some papers to the back and when I made it to the front again, a woman was standing at the counter, talking to my coworker. This woman was calm, collected, strong...There was nothing in my mind that brought me to believe she was anyone but a new patient presenting with something like cold symptoms.

It soon became clear, however, that the woman at the desk was the ambulance patient's mother. EMS, accompanied by two nurses, rushed to the registration desk and hurriedly explained that they needed mom to come back immediately to give a detailed medical history on the patient who was now unconscious.

That's right, folks...Mom didn't even go back to the child's room upon arriving to the hospital in the same ambulance. Instead, she planned on sitting in the waiting room.

A few seconds later, we received a call to let us know grandpa was on the way. My coworker and I were to let him go back as soon as he arrived.

It didn't take long for grandpa to show up. Unlike the patient's mother, the boy's grandfather was in tears, his hands were trembling, and his breathing was labored. I escorted him to the patient's room.

Staff members worked at top speeds, desperate to figure out what was going on with the little boy. While two ER doctors were lifting the boy's eyelids and checking his body for obvious signs of trauma, someone from Lab took vials of blood from the child's arm. I watched closely as the child's grandfather knelt in a prayer at the patient's bedside.

The patient's mother, on the other hand, remained at the corner of the room, with one foot out the door. She was emotionless as she stood with her arms crossed and glanced at her surroundings.

I did my best to remember we each experience emotions differently. During times of duress, some may react stoically, while others sob and hyperventilate.

I started to walk away.

"Did you give him any medicine tonight?" one of the doctors asked the patient's mother. "Or did he have access to any of your medications or toxic chemicals?"

Mom shrugged and gently shook her head.

If I said her reaction seemed to irritate the child's grandfather, it'd be a gross understatement.

Grandpa jumped up from his kneeling position and screamed at the mother, "What about all that stuff you've been shoving down his throat to make him sleep?"

The patient's mother didn't respond. She simply walked away.

This six-year-old was a patient for about a half hour before the call was made to fly him out to a children's hospital.

Police officers were involved extensively in an investigation into the child's condition, but all lab results detailing toxic substances came back clean. Mom, as far as we know, never reacted to the child's condition. Someone told me the grandfather filed an emergency guardianship request.

We don't know what happened to the boy after a three-day coma and a week-long inpatient stay at the children's facility.

Uh, if you come in and tell me your chief complaint is that you're unresponsive, you're obviously not unresponsive.

Starving for Attention

A lot of people don't seem to realize patients don't always come in from outside locations. Every now and then, floors have to transfer critically-ill patients to the ER for immediate treatment, or someone within the facility will need treatment for a fall or more extreme condition, such as a heart attack or stroke symptoms.

It was a busy day shift, but a few nurses still managed to get away from the ER to snag some lunch from the cafeteria.

Now, the last thing these two wanted to do while inhaling their lunches in a whole five minutes, I'm sure, is deal with another emergent situation. Too bad for them.

Over in the corner of the room, a frequent flyer, taking a break from visiting her OBV-admitted girlfriend, took a turn for the worse as a piece of chicken became lodged in her throat.

This woman, from what I hear, smacked her hand on the cafeteria table and flipped her full tray upside down while trying to convey to those around her that she was choking.

Our nurses over on the other side of the room took action.

The Heimlich worked too late. While the piece of unchewed chicken flew out of the woman's mouth, she wasn't breathing. CPR was started by the second nurse and someone called a code down to the switchboard operator. She, in turn, announced the code over the intercom system and paged all available personnel to the cafeteria.

Even more ER nurses rushed to the cafeteria. Doctors and nurses from other floors assisted in moving the patient to a stretcher and continuing CPR. Her shirt was removed on the way, to attach monitoring nodes and start chest compressions, and it was revealed the patient was wearing eight bras. Eight.

By the time the team made it to the ER, the patient was breathing on her own and was determined to be 'fine,' though a little 'worked up.'

Well, this patient felt the need to tell everyone what happened. She excitedly told every person from Lab, every Tech, every nurse she encountered. She made three trips to the bathroom and, on her way there and on her way back to her room, she made rounds around the nurses' station to let everyone know she was the choking patient from the cafeteria, that she stopped breathing, and it was a "horrific, traumatic experience."

Doctors decided to discharge the patient, since she seemed fine.

This irritated the patient.

Feeling she wasn't getting enough attention for what happened to her in the cafeteria, she started throwing a fit and talked about suing the hospital because nobody ever offered her another free lunch. In the middle of her breakdown, the patient flagged down a tech and begged to be checked for lice. She did everything possible to ensure all eyes were on her.

After the Nursing Supervisor negotiated with the patient, she calmed down. She didn't leave the hospital, though, after being discharged. Nope.

She took one of the free meal vouchers from the supervisor and headed back to the cafeteria.

Whatcha Got Cooking?

I often go to work in the middle of the night to take my coworkers food or just chitchat. Every now and then, something 'fun' walks in. Tonight was one of those nights.

So this young woman, I guess, decided she had enough time on her 30-minute break at an all-night diner, to drink. (That's always a good sign you're working your dream job, right?) And when I say drink, I don't mean she had a beer or two.

Nope.

Little Miss Chugalug downed a fifth of bourbon in 30 minutes and then went back to work as if nothing happened during her break.

Now, I don't know how she pulled off sobriety for even a half second, unless the alcohol didn't hit her right away. But somehow, this woman was able to navigate back to the diner's kitchen, where she was one of the cooks on duty.

How many people get hammered and think it's a good idea to try to make spaghetti at four in the morning? They usually make it through the process okay, right?

Not this woman.

In her efforts to appear sober and continue her job, she somehow set the diner's kitchen on fire.

The woman was eventually brought in for a

jail clearance. Doctors said she sustained a minor burn to her wrist and had a BAC almost six times the legal limit, but other than that, she was good to spend some time behind bars.

Stuck Up

It was the end of my shift and I was ready to go home. Time was moving in slow motion. I swore I looked at the clock at 6:32, closed my eyes for 10 minutes, and when I opened them again, it was almost 6:33.

Then walked in a crying little boy, walking with a limp alongside his laughing mother.

"What seems to be the problem this morning?" I asked, perking up at the idea that having another patient might help the shift end a bit sooner.

The boy's mother was laughing so hard tears streamed down her cheeks.

"I told him to stop hopping around like he was."

"It's not funny, mom," the boy scolded. He couldn't have been older than 10 or 11, and by the looks of it, he was in a lot of pain.

"Do we have an injury this morning?" I asked mom.

She nodded and gasped for air.

"He was doing this thing, where he was hopping from cushion to cushion on the couch, plopping down as hard as he could."

Her face was red and she needed a second to breathe.

"He had a pencil in his back pocket," she continued.

The boy hung his head.

"I kept telling him," mom chuckled, "to stop. But did he listen? Nope. He never listens."

"It's not funny, mom," the boy repeated.

"He plopped down again and stabbed himself right in the butt," mom cackled.

Hospital staff members were walking through the lobby. Most of them glanced over to the loud mom and gave me a look like they wanted some of what she had.

"So we have a puncture wound?" I asked, as I pulled up my admitting screen.

Mom took a deep breath and tried to say with a straight face, "That's not all."

I don't think she finished the first word before she was laughing again.

"What else?"

The woman looked to her child. Both of their faces were red—mom's because she couldn't breathe, and the boy's because he couldn't believe his mom was telling the world about his problem.

"It's still stuck," the mother replied.

Once I registered the patient, he was taken straight back.

And you know what? Mom wasn't joking. When her son plopped down, the dull #2 pencil punctured his right buttock, and when the force became too much, the pencil snapped almost in half, leaving a decent length of the utensil stuck.

The child didn't have to go to surgery, but it did take two ER docs an hour to remove the pencil.

Those Meddling Floors!

Some of our patients, honestly, are a few cans short of a six-pack.

For example, you and I both know not to mix bleach with ammonia. (Update: Some people have scolded me about this example. Let's say you and I know not to mix these chemicals if we think we'll be able to make drugs…I'd like to think if patients are going to try to make drugs, they'd at least Google something and learn not to mix these solutions.) And we know it's probably not the best idea to get out of the shower and try to fiddle with the outlet to figure out why the blow dryer isn't working.

And we know what happens when fugitives try to run from the cops, right?

Well, there are times when ETOH patients are transported to the hospital via ambulance, and the arresting officer arrives after finishing up at the scene of an assault, MVA, or other committed crime. Usually, this isn't a big deal.

In fact, it's only ever been a problem once.

Our newest patient that night was involved in an MVA. He was out drinking and driving, and he not only hit a parked car (which moved two houses down, it was hit with such force), but he also hit another SUV, which flipped that vehicle on its side.

Luckily, the other driver was not severely injured. She escaped the ordeal with a few bruises and superficial lacerations to her face.

Our patient, on the other hand, sustained a pretty bad hit to the back of his head. EMTs patched him up enough to transport, and he was brought it for medical attention before he was going to be carted off to the big house.

Once the patient realized the arresting officer had not arrived to the hospital yet, he had a bright idea: run.

(Because this always turns out for the best, right?)

The patient ripped out his IV, and with a bandaged head and open gown, he took off down the hall. Nurses scrambled to call security, but the patient was just too fast.

And he would have gotten away with his plan, maybe, if he hadn't slipped as he was running through the double doors that opened to the ER lobby.

The patient flew back and hit his (wanna guess?) head all over again. This time, he wasn't getting back up.

Seconds after the patient fell, the arresting officer walked inside and saw his prisoner sprawled out, surrounded by a pool of blood.

Nurses and doctors cleared the patient (again), and he was taken to jail with shackles around his wrists and ankles.

Lay it on Me

It was already a busy night and my front-desk coworker had the night off. Four chest pains came in one after the other, which was throwing us all through loops because the back was already pretty full. Patients in the waiting room were coming to the desk, demanding to know why they weren't being seen, and none of them were too understanding when I explained chest pains take precedence.

As one man was cursing at me about this 'stupid' policy, a woman hobbled in and threw herself into a wheelchair.

"What's going on right now?" I asked.

"My head hurts," she said.

Judging by her banshee shrieking, I would've guessed she had complaints of flank pain or abdominal pain.

"Might as well just come on in the waiting room," the first man said to the woman. "They call it that because you're in there so long you're just waiting to die."

Three more patients arrived and were all screaming and carrying on because they had leg pain or kidney pain or sinus pressure. Each one of the patients appeared to be trying to outdo the previous in theatrics.

When the fourth patient staggered inside, I

thought for sure she was having a heart attack. She clutched at her chest and used the wall to guide herself half-way to the registration desk.

"What's going on right now?" I asked.

She pouted.

Pou-ted.

Stuck out her lower lip and frowned.

I stood and moved forward. "Let's put you in a wheelchair."

"I can't," she said.

"We need to, especially if you can't walk without assistance."

"I can't."

"What's hurting right now?"

"My head's going to explode," she said.

Realizing the patient wasn't going to sit in the wheelchair I had grabbed, I made my way back to my desk.

"What's your name?"

She screamed at me, "I can't do this."

"We have to get you in the system before we can do anything."

This woman...

I kid you not...

I have to start my sentences that way because that's about how I was dealing with my patience at that moment.

This woman dropped to her knees very slowly

and gently, placed her palms on the floor, and proceeded to lie down on the rug in front of the registration desk. She then rolled back and forth and screamed at the top of her lungs.

I called the Charge Nurse.

"Who's doing that screaming?" were his first words to me.

I explained, "This woman said her head feels like it's going to explode."

"Just go ahead and get her registered," he said. "I'll try to figure out which of us isn't knee deep in Cath Lab admits and try to send someone up in a minute."

"That's the thing," I hurriedly added. "She keeps saying she can't answer questions or sit in a wheelchair. She's on the floor right now."

The Charge Nurse paused and then laughed with a scoff, "Are you kidding me right now? Is that her, rolling around in front of the desk?"

"Ye—."

"Is she taking her shirt off? Oh, wow. This woman's taking her shirt off in the lobby. What in the world?"

I could hear the doc in back talking as he moved closer to the Charge Nurse in order to view the monitor displaying footage from the lobby security camera.

"We'll send someone out right now to help you."

While I was waiting for someone to come up

from the back, security saw the ordeal and came out to try to help the patient into a wheelchair.

She repeated, "I can't," louder and louder each time they attempted to reason with her, so they backed off.

Finally, a few nurses came out and tried to gather information from the woman.

She still wouldn't say anything other than, "I can't," and she refused to get up off the floor.

"I need something for the pain," she begged. "I need Dilaudid."

Several of us may or may not have rolled our eyes at this moment.

"You need to get in a wheelchair if you want us to help you."

"Didn't you hear me?" the woman shouted. "I need Dilaudid."

For sure, I thought the woman was going to pull out an excuse like, 'My doctor from six counties away said I'm allergic to everything but Dilaudid. I'd tell you to call him, but a UFO took over his town and he doesn't have a working phone because his ex-wife took it in the divorce. So I guess you'll have to trust me.'

"And didn't you hear me?" the nurse, short on patience, retorted. "Get in the wheelchair or we can't help you."

The patient stood with no assistance and *walked* to the back, where she was placed in a room. (This did nothing to calm the people in the waiting room—when they saw another patient was taken back, I heard a bunch of groans.) Her husband came in a few seconds later and gave me her information for registration.

"I'm sorry," he said. "I could hear her outside."

"Does she get headaches like this a lot?"

The husband laughed. "She has a cold. She's the biggest wimp I know when it comes to being sick."

Throughout the patient's short stay, she was fairly demanding. I heard her shout a few times, and right before she was discharged, she came back to the registration desk in her hospital gown to ask where she could find a vending machine.

The woman's 'rather bizarre' behavior was noted in her chart.

Oh, and she reported all of our shift for not getting her to the back soon enough and for not making her comfortable.

At least once a week we see a parent bring his/her child in for something superficial (runny nose, red toe, burping excessively), spend most of his/her time outside (smoking, texting, talking to everyone and anyone), and ask more times for a note to get out of work than they ask anything about his/her child's discharge instructions.

Not Full of...

Registration received a very...*odd* phone call one night.

A man called in to ask if he should be seen by a doctor for a, um, problem he experienced following intercourse.

According to the frightened-sounding man, he and his wife were engaging in intercourse and everything was 'going okay.' When he ejaculated, however, 'something weird happened.'

That something weird?

Our caller said his face went numb, he lost consciousness for what his wife estimated was about five to ten seconds, and he, uh...

The man voided his bowels.

While he was still on top of his wife.

Unconscious.

We transferred the call back to one of the nurses, pretty sure it was a prank, but slightly unsure, as the caller seemed sincere in his fear and embarrassment.

The man didn't come in that night, so if he was serious, he obviously didn't feel it was that much of an emergency.

Yes, people really do call the ER and ask to be transferred to 911.

In fact, it just happened again two nights ago.

All for One and One for All?

At this hospital, if you present with a chief complaint of chest pain, a number of questions are asked to determine severity of the situation. Some of these questions, usually asked by Triage are:

How old are you?

Can you please point to where it hurts?

Does your pain radiate anywhere?

Have you experienced a heart problem before?

During times when colds are going around, we often ask if the patient has been coughing, especially if he/she is younger and states he/she has not experienced a heart problem before.

When a teenager arrived at the desk with three of her friends and told me she had chest pain, I asked if she'd had a heart problem, to which she stated no. She said she had been coughing, so I registered her. Because she was the next patient and we only had one patient in the back, I knew this would not disrupt the time frame in which nurses were required to perform an EKG.

Well, though I tried to explain this to the patient, she and her friends developed some 'holier than thou' attitude and decided I wasn't good enough to talk to. I tried three times to tell them a nurse was on the way up, but each time, one or more of the girls yelled at me.

I could hear the nurse talking as she walked nearer to the registration desk.

All four girls, however, were long gone. See, one of them needed to go to the bathroom.

They all decided to file into the one-commode public restroom.

The nurse rolled her eyes when I explained the situation. We waited 10 minutes for the young ladies to emerge from the restroom.

And, I swear, when the girls came out of the bathroom, the patient's hair had gone from long and flowing to a messy braid that curled over her shoulder, and two of the girls were sporting fresh layers of lipstick.

Oh...The patient was fine. She was discharged with heartburn.

A Prayer Before Work

"Please don't let some drunk old man wave his penis around at me today. It would also be great if I'm not groped, asked out, or harassed.

If someone has to throw up, may it please be in the Eme-Bag and not on 1.) me, 2.) my desk, or 3.) where it will hold up the line when we're super busy.

I'd really appreciate it if I don't have to smell C. Diff today, and I know it's a lot to ask, but maybe you can fix this so most of the patients either bathe or wear deodorant today.

Please keep our department safe from patients with 1.) complaints against the organization and/or its staff, 2.) mentally unstable patients, 3.) that one butthole doctor with a god complex, and/or 4.) addicts.

If someone vomits, bleeds, urinates, defecates, or transfers bodily fluids onto my $60 scrubs, may I be blessed to have a clean set in my locker and not have to wear the mismatched donor scrubs that make me look like I'm 12 and dressing in my great-grandmother's clothes.

Now, I know there's not a carry-in today, but I left my lunch on the kitchen counter, so if someone could maybe bring in some food, that'd be awesome. I am also not opposed to drinking anything spiked with alcohol during my shift, because who would I be to turn away one of your blessings?

Please aide me in practicing patience, tolerance, and understanding. I'm sure you've noticed I could also use some help with biting my tongue, keeping sarcastic comments to myself, and not walking out when I'm frustrated. Please bless our patients and when I'm confronted with difficult patients, please allow me to only reply with a sweetly presented, "Bless your heart."

If you could help me out in these areas, I would be forever grateful. Look forward to another session when I have to come back in sixteen hours."

Welcome to the Emergency Room, where you'll be first if you're the worst!

Sorry it's Not What You Wanted

With Christmas right around the corner, everyone in the ER was preparing. Holiday decorations were up on most of the doors in the back, someone put up garland in a heart rhythm pattern along the corridor wall, and up front, the window behind the registration desk was decked out with handmade decorations and stockings we decorated over a few not-so-busy shifts.

Along with the decoration preparations, a lot of us had just finished shopping for stocking stuffers and our secret Santa gifts. My awesome coworker decided to buy novelty gifts for everyone on the registration staff, as well as distribute novelty gifts to the nurses and doctors in back. She found a bulk package of badge holders online, but what she was really excited to hand out to everyone were these nifty little pens that were shaped like syringes. Each pen contained an outer cylinder of fake 'medication,' in various colors and were shipped in a cardboard container that resembled a vial holder.

Overall, the week was going well, which we all knew was a sign that all holy hell was about to break loose.

And, oh, did it ever on one of the overnight shifts, of course.

For three hours straight, my coworker and I were slammed. In the back, they were short two nurses and the two they called in lived at least 30 minutes away. Everyone was sweaty, hungry, and slightly aggravated that the universe picked our shift to make up for all of those peaceful shifts throughout the week.

Just as the last bed in back was filled by a genuinely sick patient, one of our frequent flyers stumbled inside.

Security recognized the man and came out immediately.

"I need help," he pleaded.

"We'll get you signed in," I said. "Go ahead and sign the consent form, okay?"

"Help me," he blubbered.

"Sign the form for me," I repeated. "I just got you in the system. It's going to be a little bit before we can get you in the back."

The man broke out in a full wail.

"Bad meth," he cried. "It was bad meth."

Every single time he did meth, he came to us in the same condition: remorseful, sobbing, and repetitive in his requests.

"We'll have you sit on the bench," I told the man. "And we'll tell the Charge Nurse you're here."

The man didn't listen. He paced in circles and fell a few times, all while yelling, "Somebody help me."

All of the nurses in the back were busy. We had four traumas on the board, two stemis, and one DID (died in department).

Security attempted to direct the addict to the bench, but when he refused to follow directions, they simply allowed him to wander around to avoid some of his violent outbursts.

Patients continued flooding inside, trying to steer clear of the obviously-impaired man.

My coworker and I continued our jobs.

You know, I really didn't think much of it when my personal ink pen ran dry. Right after I tossed the empty pen in the trash can, I dug through my purse for another pen. The only one I could find was the novelty pen she put in my stocking, a 'syringe' filled with bright blue 'medication.'

Still not thinking much about it, I continued scribbling on some paperwork and set the pen down on the edge of the desk as I labeled pages for our latest patient.

Before I even realized what was happening, the meth-man rushed to the desk and swiped my pen.

I didn't say anything. Security started to move toward the man, but he *finally* sat on the bench and was quiet for the first time since he'd arrived.

We all watched the man as he fiddled with the pen and held it up to the light to get a better view of the liquid inside.

"What is this? Is it good?" he asked.

I wanted to laugh. It was so hard not to.

Instead, I bit my lip.

The man, in so much pain from a bad high, yet so desperate for another fix, tried to insert the pen's 'needle' in a vein on his arm. When he couldn't get the 'needle' to stick him, he looked confused, inspected the pen, and then said with a laugh, "Holy [long string of expletives], it's a pen."

Patient Quiz:

If you have asthma and COPD, yet only have enough money to purchase either your inhaler or a pack of cigarettes, which would you choose?

<u>Drastic Measures</u>

For some reason, some patients can't seem to grasp the concept of the fullness of waiting room in relation to the number of occupied beds in back.

Sometimes I want to say, "Can we just get this straight? If I could send you to the back right now, I would. I'm sure the nurses would gladly treat you and send you on your not-so-merry way just so you'll stop yelling at everyone."

I can't say that, though, and there's nothing I can do to make the process go any faster.

Patients in the waiting room sometimes think they can.

A few times a week, we see that one patient who's able to walk in, but as soon as his feet hit the lobby floor, he needs a wheelchair—which he'll fall out of and onto the waiting room floor about three times, all while he's screaming and moaning, just to see if it will work.

A woman may come in with 'severe' abdominal pain, yet be fine enough to drink a bottle of soda and eat a family-size bag of chips while she argues with another patient over which channel should be on the waiting room TV. As soon as a doctor or nurse walks by, that woman will be in the most pain ev-er...at least until nobody rushes over and says, "Oh, let me take you straight back."

You know, after seeing this patient, I can honestly say I've seen it all in the desperate attempts to get to the back faster.

I came in a bit early to cover for a sick coworker, and dang, did I regret it. On the way to work, I had to pull over for three ambulances. When you live in a moderately-small town and there's one hospital, you don't really get a chance to hope those emergency vehicles are taking people elsewhere.

At work, I couldn't find a close place to park. In fact, there were so many cars in the lot that people had taken to making up their own parking spaces.

As I walked inside, I passed two empty police cars and could see through the open waiting room blinds there were only two empty chairs.

I can't recall a time I've ever said more curse words before I even got in the building than while I was in it than that night.

All staff members were a mess. Some of the registration people were close to tears. Security had their hands full with helping the local PD with two patients under the influence of who-knows-what. Registered patients were wandering the lobby and yelling at their kids and texting and eating and everything else they could possibly do to pass the time. A few of them came to the desk to ask how long it'd take to be seen.

One woman in particular caught our eyes. Several times, she approached the desk but wouldn't say anything.

When I asked my coworkers what her main complaint was, I was told she was there for dental pain and wanted to be seen as soon as possible.

Well, in a pile of patients presenting with lacerations and flank pain and SOB and jaundice, we knew dental pains were likely to be...not overlooked, but placed lower on the scale of importance set in place by the Triage rules.

After 45 minutes, the patient approached the desk.

"I need to be seen now," she demanded.

"I'm sorry, but people are moving as quickly as possible, based on receiving adequate treatment."

Well, you know how it goes when you try to be all professional...you make people mad.

This lady, was apparently already mad.

She reached into this tiny little purse she had hanging off her shoulder and pulled out something that I thought looked like a knife. I didn't get the best look, and I wasn't really expecting what she did, so I guess I didn't pay the best attention.

I kind of looked away from the lobby for a few seconds, maybe to look at my computer screen or something. At the time, what I was doing seemed more important, but now I realize it was insignificant compared to that evening's events.

"Do I have to be dying to be seen by a doctor?" the woman shouted.

Everyone looked up then, just in time to see the patient plunge a sharp object through her loose floral dress and into her belly.

Someone yelled for Triage and I stat-paged security. They removed a letter opener from the patient's possession and assisted with transporting the patient to a trauma room that had just been labeled clean as the woman harmed herself.

It took a while to get the patient fixed up. In the end, she didn't mention her dental pain.

She asked to be transferred to another hospital.

So, um, if you know that your allergy to something results in anaphylactic shock and you don't have an EpiPen on hand, it's probably not a smart idea to 'try it, just to see if [you're] still allergic to it.'

But what do I know? I'm just the registration clerk.

A Blessing and a Curse

This story as difficult to write as it was to experience.

In the emergency room, you are constantly surrounded by the good and bad. I've seen miracles and I've seen heartaches. This one was a bit of both.

Five minutes before my shift ended, I found myself anxiously tapping my nails on the desk, wondering where my relief was and when he would arrive. It hadn't really been a trying night. In fact, it was fairly slow, I guess. Nothing too exciting happened.

I saw a car pull up in front of the entrance and a man ran inside.

Before I could say anything, he blurted out, "Wife. Labor. Need help."

Two just-on-shift ER nurses heard the man and rushed outside. They were snapping on blue gloves as they approached the car.

I called the back and explained to the day-shift Charge Nurse what was going on. She came up front with two more nurses.

Just as that group headed toward the door, both of the first nurses ran inside, holding bloodied newborns to their chests.

Instead of the entire second group running

outside, the Charge Nurse ordered the already-running pack behind her to grab a bed from the back.

There wasn't much I could do at this point, other than watch and try to communicate to the Unit Clerk what was happening. I made sure to keep the double doors open so the crew could move mom inside quickly.

When the nurses rolled mom's stretcher inside, her sweatpants were soaked in blood and she appeared to be unconscious. Her husband was crying as he followed everyone into the back.

He kept repeating in a panic, "She pushed both of them out while I was inside. She's only twenty-six weeks."

I started receiving frantic calls from multiple nurses to do anything I could to get the patients—all three of them—in the system as soon as possible. Mom and one of her daughters were receiving oxygen and were being prepped to go to OB.

One of her daughters.

While both girls were born alive, one passed away as soon as she was taken into a room. The other was being transferred to a hospital with a NICU as soon as she could be stabilized.

According to some of the chitchat around the department that day, the parents knew one of the girls would be born with fatal physical defects. They prepared themselves for that as much as they could. They couldn't, however, know that the baby would die in womb. This seemed to set off a reaction in her body that sent her into premature labor.

The patient and her daughter survived.

When you work in the ER, some common words and phrases mean something else entirely.

March Madness: Well, we're still trying to recover from December, January, and February Madness.

Thirsty Thursdays: Double to triple amount of ETOH patients.

Spring Break: Oh, dear Lord, no. Please, all of you, just go HOME! Also known as: just because your mother didn't specifically teach you that it's a bad idea to jump from a rooftop into a shallow pool of beer doesn't mean it's still not a bad idea.

Snow Day: Screw you for posting pictures of that 'beautiful' snow as you sip cocoa. I can tell you from experience that it wasn't so beautiful when I fell in it three times while trying to scrape the nine-inches of ice off my windshield so I could go listen to 14-hours of call lights.

Weekend: Just another day. We don't get the luxury of having a lot of these off.

Super Bowl Sunday: One of those rare occasions we can predict when we'll be busy, what time 'business' will slow, when it will pick up again, and also get a good idea of just how drunk our patients will be when they get here...all based on that same little box you're watching.

ER Secret:

There are times it smells so bad in the ER that anyone can fart and blame it on that little old lady with diarrhea in room 12.

Every Parent's Nightmare

A new mom showed up when the ER lobby and waiting room were packed. She pushed her way to the front of the line and interrupted us as we were registering a patient and dealing with phone calls regarding an emergency on ICU.

"Ma'am," I said, "I'll need you to step back until—."

"I need help," she yelled.

The woman held up one car seat and then another. I never even saw her bring them in.

"I dropped them," she frantically stated. "They're only five days old."

The triage nurse heard the commotion and told me to go ahead and register the newborns. She stepped back in her office and notified the Charge Nurse of two incoming Ped traumas.

Mom was hysterical and had to be given a shot of Ativan to calm down.

She explained she was carrying the twins through the kitchen so she could grab a bottle from a warmer, when she tripped over her dog. She fell forward and tried to twist as she went down, but it all happened too fast. Both babies' heads hit the tile kitchen floor, and mom sprained her ankle.

It didn't take long to determine both infants sustained skull fractures and one had a brain bleed.

Don't fret. Both children made a speedy recovery.

Do you ever stop to think about how much money could be made if someone could invent a common sense injection?

"You Were Stabbed Where?"

It had been moderately slow all night, and I had just gotten through joking with my coworker about how the universe seems to sense when she leaves and I'm alone. See, that's when all hell breaks loose.

My coworker laughed and told me it wouldn't be all that bad. She was scheduled another two hours, so we'd do our best to keep the flow to a minimum.

And then, since nothing was going on, she went to the back to take a break and talk to some of the nurses.

As soon as my coworker was out of sight, two patients signed in and another man came inside for a wheelchair, which told me the obvious: there was a third patient outside.

I registered the two patients at the desk and answered three phone calls in a span of four minutes.

Just as I was getting off the phone with ICU, the man from earlier wheeled in an OB patient.

There I was, trying to quickly register a woman as she was having contractions that were a minute apart, when another man came in screaming.

"My brother took some bad drugs. I'm bringing him in now."

I've never typed faster on that work keyboard than I was then, trying to wrap up the OB patient's chart. I dialed the operator and paged an orderly just as the screaming man wheeled in his brother.

I directed the OB patient and her husband to the waiting room and waved for the screaming man to bring his brother to the desk.

The man in the wheelchair was drooling and his head was bobbing. Security saw this and came to the lobby in an instant.

Thankfully, one of the security guards notified the Charge Nurse of the patient in the wheelchair. I scrambled to get him registered.

To make everything just a little more hectic, two women ran through the doors hollering about drugs and alcohol and who knows what else. One of the women said the man in the wheelchair was her boyfriend. She thought he snorted cocaine that was laced with something else.

And then she said she needed a rape kit performed because she was drugged.

I can't quite describe what I was feeling in that moment. What I can tell you, however, is that there comes a time when I become completely overwhelmed by what is occurring around me that I can't move, except to let out a nervous laugh that, in itself, screams, 'Are you freaking kidding me?!'

The security guard came back from speaking with the Charge Nurse, and once I explained about the drug-man's wife, he simply nodded, spun around on his heels, and went to the back again.

Meanwhile, the mother of the man in the wheelchair was on her cellphone, threatening someone.

So...stay with me.

Two patients with whatever complaints...One labor check. One overdose. One rape kit. A mom yelling at someone.

"Okay," I stated, "you're both registered. Nurses are heading up here right now."

"You two," I said to the brother and mother, "can hang out in the waiting room. It generally takes the nurses a few minutes to get the patient adjusted in the room."

"No," mom argued. "We're not done."

"Not done?" I asked, with raised brows.

"I got stabbed," the standing brother said, like he was just announcing something ordinary.

And this is where I just lost it.

My head whipped around so fast I could give that chick from The Exorcist a run for her money.

"You were stabbed?" I exclaimed. "Where?"

"At the park," shrugged our Jethro Bodine-Grand Theft Auto mashup.

I shook my head and am pretty sure my eyes shook from side to side, too. That's how overwhelmed I was at that moment.

"No," I said. "Where? Where were you

stabbed?"

He seemed confused.

I took a deep breath and knew I had to break it down.

"Where on your body were you stabbed? Show me where you were stabbed."

"The pit."

"You were stabbed where?" I laughed nervously.

The man rolled up the sleeve of his tee shirt, lifted his arm, and showed me his mangled armpit. As soon as the wound wasn't being held together by the pressure of his arm pressed against his body, it gushed blood.

"They stabbed me in the armpit. It hurts pretty bad."

I nodded and put my fingers to my temple.

"Whoa," said the security guard, in shock. "What's going on now?"

In a calm voice, with a heavy touch of disbelief, I said to him, almost as if I was skeptical about the situation, "He got stabbed in the armpit. Like, for real. Someone stabbed him in the armpit."

Well, there went the security guard for the third time.

No sooner than I registered the stab wound did my coworker come back from her break.

She took one look at the people in the waiting

room, the OB patient and her husband trying to breathe through contractions, the man in the wheelchair, the crying wife, the bloody brother, and the mom—who was still shouting at someone.

"What happened while I was gone?" she said with wide eyes.

I shrugged and said in a broken voice, "The universe. It knows."

Working the night shift is great...you get the feeling of a hangover without drinking, and you never quite know what day it is when you wake up from a nap.

<u>Seeing Stars</u>

A lot of people dream about meeting celebrities. We were discussing this at work one night, and we all came to the conclusion that if it ever happens, we'd all prefer it did not happen at work.

Luckily for us, not too many celebrities are ever going to roll through our tiny town.

Well, there was one...

I first saw this woman at shift change. It was another one of those mornings when my relief was running late, leaving me with five new patients at once, all determined to scream louder than the patient ahead.

Anyway, this patient was doubled over in a wheelchair. She moaned and groaned and any attempt to learn what was wrong with her was met by shrieks.

I turned to the woman's friend.

"What's happening with her?"

The friend didn't seem too interested as he played with his cellphone.

"Don't know. Said her stomach hurts."

The friend then walked away, still on his cell phone.

As I was registering the (brand new to our

system) patient, I thought I saw the woman's friend waving his phone around, but I didn't think much of it. I honestly thought he was trying to find service.

Well, I left work and that was that.

I thought so, anyway.

When I went back to work the next night, I learned the same patient had been back three times since I clocked out. This wasn't a huge surprise; some patients return several times in short periods if their pain persists.

"There are some problems with twelve," one of my coworkers said, pulling me aside. "Nobody's allowed to go back."

I shrugged it off. "Okay."

"Do you even know who that is?"

"Yeah," I replied. "I was here when she first came in."

My coworker shook his head. "I mean, do you know her?"

"No."

"You haven't heard of her before?"

How many times did I have to say no?

"She's famous."

"Can't be that famous," I muttered.

"No," he argued. "She's maybe not famous here, but she's a country singer. She has videos and everything."

I shrugged again. "Okay."

He dragged me to the computer and typed in the patient's stage name. Thousands of results returned from Google, including pictures of the patient on stage in front of giant crowds, videos of the singer receiving standing ovations.

"She's here," he said. "That has to mean something, right?"

"She's just a normal person," I answered. "Maybe she's here to visit family or something."

Right around that time, we heard screaming from the back and security high-tailed it to 12.

The commotion was unreal. We could hear nurses barking orders and the patient's visitors arguing with security. They were still bickering when security escorted them out.

"You can't do this," yelled the same man I'd seen on my last shift. His cell phone was in the air, and I could see the screen for a split second. He was recording everything.

"What you were doing is against HIPAA," security explained.

"I need this," the man responded. "We're almost finished with it."

Our guard raised his brow. "Finished with what?"

"Nothing," the man said, realizing his mistake.

"Finished with what?" the guard asked again. "Do I need to call in the cops?"

The man looked shocked and put his hands up.

"No, man. No. It's nothing bad. We're not

harming anyone."

"Then what did you mean?"

Everyone was watching the argument at this point.

And then someone else chimed in.

The patient emerged from the double doors, wearing a hospital gown.

"It was my idea," she said. "We're trying to make a music video."

"You've got to be sh—," I started, under my breath.

The patient continued, "We needed authenticity."

Our guard shook his head in stupor. "For real?"

"Yes," the patient nodded.

No amount of hometown awards or crowds' ovations or votes for newcomer to the country music industry (I don't know if that's even an award she won, by the way, so let's not jump to conclusions) could save the patient from this situation.

She apologized profusely to security and to nurses in the back for the 'scene' she caused. There was nothing she could say, however, to take back all the wasted resources and time spent treating a patient with false claims. Our patient admitted she was faking her condition and endured sticks and pokes and an IV for the 'sake of offering fans reality.'

I don't follow celebrities a whole lot, and I don't even know if that's what you'd consider our former patient. In some respect, I suppose she's one to many, and from what I saw from her videos and acting abilities, she obviously possesses a persistent, raw talent. My coworkers told me, not long after the 'session,' the patient posted 'art' to her social media page.

The 'art,' I hear, was a picture of the patient while she was in room 12.

Welcome to the ER, where your 'worst day ever' is our everyday.

No Massive Parties at the ER

A mother brought in a toddler to be seen for fussiness and abdominal pain. Mom seemed genuinely concerned about her child, so we didn't think anything of the visit.

Well, over the span of about an hour, mom's concern for the child seemed to dwindle. She must have gone in and out about 10 times to smoke and talk on her cell phone.

"How much longer is this going to take?" she asked me.

I told her what I knew, which was that the tracking board was still showing the child had six open tests and only two had been completed. It would probably be a while longer.

Mom muttered something about it 'being Friday night' and walked back outside. A few minutes later, she returned to her kid's room.

Some time passed. More people started coming in. I didn't think too much about anything, really, except taking care of patients and finishing my reports.

I had to take a few documents to the Unit Clerk and passed a nurse as she was on the way to the toddler's room. The child was crying rather loudly. We just figured the baby was still feeling ill.

Before I could make it to the Unit Clerk's area, the toddler's nurse came out into the hallway, holding the patient.

"Kerry," she hissed to me.

"Huh?"

"Did you see his mom go back outside?"

I shook my head. "It's been a while."

"I gave her a bottle for him, but it's sitting on the table, and it's cold. That was about thirty minutes ago. Can you see if she's outside?"

Everything else came to a halt. Paperwork had to wait. New patients had to wait.

I went outside, but mom was nowhere around. When I reported this back to the toddler's nurse, she notified security and they started a low-key search for the patient's mother.

A half hour later, the search ending with no results and the police were notified. And, coincidentally, shortly after they arrived, a man arrived. He identified himself as the toddler's father.

"My ex sent me a text," he said. He was panting and his face was red. "Is my son here?"

According to the man, who lived an hour away, received a text from his ex, stating she 'couldn't wait around forever' and wanted to attended a 'massive' party. So, like any great mom would do, she left her child at the hospital and was arrested at the party for neglect of a minor.

The toddler's dad, from what we heard from

law enforcement at a later date, took mom back to court and gained full custody. Mom, I guess, was in and out of jail for petty crimes afterward.

I don't say, "goodbye," to frequent flyers. I say, "See you later." My logic in this is knowing they'll be back soon.

It took about two minutes and the patient repeating 19 times that he thought he had 'minion-itis' to realize he meant 'meningitis.'

<u>Don't Fix It</u>

Two college kids approached the registration desk at four in the morning.

"How can I help you?" asked my coworker.

One of them stepped forward. "I need to see a doctor. I have this weird rash...down there."

He pointed to his genitals, of course, and lost color in his face when he did.

My coworker registered the patient.

"If you want to have a seat, they'll come get you as soon as they're ready," she instructed.

The second guy stepped to the desk.

"Hey," he said. "Do they charge for everything here?"

My coworker thought and then nodded.

"So you think they'd charge me for an x-ray, even if I didn't actually want to see a doctor in the emergency room?"

"Well," she responded, "it's four in the morning and the only place to be seen here right now is through the ER. And, yes, they charge for x-rays."

"Dang," he muttered.

He lifted the sleeve of his jacket and plopped his arm up on the counter.

"See," he said, "I hit my wrist on the door when we were leaving."

He turned it. "I'm pretty sure it's broken. It hurts when I turn it."

My coworker and I both blankly stared at the young man for a second.

"Do you think it's broken?" asked the man.

"I can't give a medical opinion," she replied, "but I can tell you from experience that if you broke it, it'd hurt a little more than you're letting on."

The patient rotated his wrist as far left as it would go and he winced.

"You mean like this?"

"Go sit down and we'll call you when your friend is next," I chimed in, fighting laughter.

The man returned a few hours later and said his girlfriend told him his wrist 'looked pretty bad' and he needed an x-ray because she was a second-year nursing student and was 'pretty sure' it was broken.

It wasn't broken.

It wasn't even cracked.

He simply had a bruise.

Hate on me if you must, but I have to say: I don't want his girlfriend to be my nurse until she's gotten some years on her.

Florence Nightingale Pledge

As far as I'm aware, I didn't mention anything about this next story in either of the other books. At the time, it was too fresh. But in today's world, maybe it's about time to tell the story, to honor an amazing wife and mother, to share a message, and to bring attention to some of the strength and tact healthcare providers possess and display.

One of our overnight shifts didn't start so well. It was busy and the 7a-7p, 7p-7a, and 11a-11p nurses were working overtime together, scrambling to get a surreal amount of patients admitted to floors.

So, you know, at first, when one of the nurses didn't show up on time, it was sort of shrugged off. The woman had three kids and was just talking about how her husband had some kind of head cold. She was probably stuck dealing with some small hiccup at home.   Nobody bothered calling her. Nobody really did much of anything beside joke around that she was going to get the first few patients of the overnight shift to make up for what the others were handling.

And then a half hour passed.

Things started slowing down and people started worrying.

They called her cell.

No answer.

They couldn't reach her husband.

The home phone kept switching over to the answering machine.

Then a call came over the ambulance radio.

EMS called in an MVA but didn't give all the details. They simply said a driver was being transported to our facility. Nobody said anything else. They didn't mention names, ages, locations...nothing.

Our people were antsy. The Charge Nurse called in the Nursing Supervisor and two security guards. All four had a little pow-wow in the consult room.

As they were speaking, EMS arrived with the MVA patient.

We were all relieved to see the patient was not our coworker, was not our nurse. Instead, this was a man, a stranger. He was beat up, bloody, and he needed help.

Now, I don't care if I'm the registration clerk, the doctor, the CEO of the hospital, the Tech, part of Lab, or the janitor who scrubs puke off the chair or blood off the surgery room floors. I don't know how it works at other hospitals, and I don't know how other people think, but in this industry, every single worker has an obligation to show compassion to any patient, regardless of skin color, religion, sexual orientation, income, education level, or any other aspect that distinguishes one human being from another on a caste system chart.

That is why the MVA patient received care from four nurses, two doctors, had registration at his side asking if he wanted to notify anyone on his NOK (next of kin) list, and had x-ray waiting to make sure he was okay.

A while after the patient was in the hospital's care, a few state troopers arrived, with a few local PD in tow. Unfortunately, they had some bad news.

Our coworker wasn't absent from work because she was dealing with a family matter. She was missing from work because as she was driving in, a drunk driver crossed the median, hit her vehicle head on, and then tried to flee from the scene. The nurse, a beautiful, caring, funny, smart, bubbly, Godly woman was ejected from her minivan—the one she was so proud of because she said it was just another symbol of her role as a busy mother—and thrown 20-something feet. She was pronounced dead at the scene.

By now, you've probably figured out what we were just figuring out.

Yes, our MVA patient was the drunk driver. His BAC was five times the legal limit, and he was tied to a sexual predator case.

Now, how do you continue to offer care to someone who killed your best friend? How do you still compassionately treat a person you want to start hitting and never stop? How do you stand over a man you'd see on the front page news and tell your husband or wife or grandmother you couldn't even believe could do something so heinous, yet suture his lacerations?

I can't answer that question because I just don't know how it's done. I don't know how our nurses talked to grief counselors in the consult room, yet walked right back into that patient's room and made sure he didn't die, too. I don't know how they cared that his catheter bag was full or that he needed just a bit more medication to keep his heart rate steady. When he started to crash, I don't know how they could look at this man as anything but a killer.

But they did.

And you know what? These people do it EVERY. SINGLE. DAY. These nurses took an oath to provide the best care to every patient, no matter if that patient is a drug dealer, a child molester, a rapist, a cop-killer, a poor man who was just trying to protect the only home he had, a priest, someone HIV positive...there are no limits when you come to the hospital as a patient.

Now, I'm not saying this patient wasn't on the receiving end of the largest-gauge needles. I'm not saying maybe it didn't take the doctor just a *little* longer to order more pain medication.

If that happened, I can't really say.

All I know is, at the end of the night, the patient was stabilized and the decision was made to transfer him to a different facility.

It is possible, I've learned, to care about a person's life but disagree with a decision he or she has made or an action he or she has performed.

And nobody can do that better than a nurse.

Woman called 911 and was brought in via ambulance for an out of body experience.

I'm sure a positive PCP level on the blood test had juuuuuust a little bit to do with all of that.

<u>Helpful Items to Bring to the ER:</u>

- Medication list, including your daily dosage

   If you are traveling, ALWAYS carry an up-to-date list.

- A list of your surgeries, especially if you can't remember/are visiting a new facility

- Phone numbers for each of the following:

   1.) A next of kin

   2.) A ride home, provided your NOK is not nearby

- Cell phone charger

- A small amount of cash or a debit/credit card is advised, just in case you are discharged and need to pay for a prescription on the way home

- A friend—I watched a man sit in the waiting room for six hours after he received a pain shot. He couldn't legally drive home.

To be completely honest, I can't think of a single other item you would **need** in an emergent situation. We have people at the registration desk with three bags of clothes for a cough, while a cancer patient can't remember his what medication he takes.

A Prayer for After Work

"Please be with me as I consume a few adult beverages. My goal is to not vomit in the back yard, so if you could help with that, I would greatly appreciate it. I know it's a lot to ask, but I'd also be grateful if you could make sure I'm not hungover, too.

By the way, please don't let them call me in early."

If this is the worst ER ever, WHY do you keep coming back?

__Child Protection__

I had just arrived at work and didn't even have a chance to put my purse down or take my coat off before patients waiting in the lobby flooded the desk when they set sights on an extra registration person at the desk.

Unfortunately, due to our layout, we can only offer service to one family at a time.

So, as I settled in, a mother with a young child in her arms approached the desk.

"He doesn't want to move," was the mother's chief complaint regarding her child. The young boy was draped over his mother's shoulder, and a man stood next to her.

My coworker continued registering the patient, and I didn't think much of it. The little boy looked fairly tired and didn't move much, but we see a lot of that, the later the evening grows.

Well, when Triage showed up for the patient, it became clear that there was something severely wrong. When the nurse asked the boy's mother to place the patient in a wheelchair, the child couldn't hold his head up.

"Did you know about this?" he asked me.

"I would have called you immediately if I knew," I replied.

The child was taken to a room and we didn't

hear anything for a while.

Then, out of the blue, a nurse from the back approached me.

"DCFS is on its way," she said quietly.

It didn't take any sort of special skill to deduce the agency was called for the young boy.

"Do you know what happened?" I asked.

The nurse shook her head. "No. Yes. I don't know."

She explained, "The boy shows evidence of abuse: bruising, healed fractures, healing fractures. But then he told x-ray that someone hits him. He won't say who, though."

For more than an hour, we all had to pretend that we knew nothing. And really, that wasn't such a far stretch because we didn't know a lot. Mom and step-dad kept going out to smoke. They seemed like nice people, and the mom's sister dropped off a baby with the couple.

DCFS showed up a while later. And this is when things started to get a bit...well, things weren't great.

At first, mom and step-dad took the initial line of investigation okay. They weren't thrilled, of course, but they were cooperative.

But then the little boy was marked as an admit to PEDs and a few calls were made.

Both of the adults were asked to speak with DCFS in the empty waiting room, away from the children.

I can't even explain all of the details because everything happened so quickly, but before I knew it, the child of the little boy was screaming and someone was walking outside with the child dropped off a bit earlier. According to DCFS, the child was not to be in the father's custody at all, and the agent stated the police were notified, but the baby's mother declined to press charges.

I wondered how the patient's mother would react when it came down to her own child, given how she responded to her husband's baby.

The agent began explaining there was evidence of abuse found with our patient. Surprisingly (to me, anyway), neither parent reacted in a way I expected. Both adults were calm and tearful. They spoke in front of DCFS to come up with an idea of who could abuse their child.

But when the agent stated the parents were banned from visiting the admitted child without a nurse's consent, they flipped.

Mom threw a magazine across the waiting room. Our patient's step-dad stormed outside and chain smoked.

"You have no jurisdiction over when I see my child, especially in a hospital," the mother screamed at the social worker.

Ummmm....That's not exactly true, from what I was told. But that wasn't even the worst part.

The social worker took security with her when she informed the patient's mother and step-father that a judge signed a court order removing the child from their custody.

Still, they weren't as livid as I expected.

Both adults began calling family members responsible for the child's care within the time frame our nurses estimated.

As it turns out, the parents were *not* responsible for the abuse. Their son was taken to a woman every Wednesday for the entire day. Investigators discovered the woman had not only beaten our patient, but was responsible for abusing eight other minors.

When I'm working a bad shift, I wonder how anyone ever figured out how to work a catheter.

And then I'm just glad I wasn't one of the first hundred practice patients.

Healthcare worker hangover:
"I should register & ask for a banana bag."

A male patient presented with the chief complaint, "My brain is on fire."

These are about the only words he spoke during his visit.

Lab results showed the patient tested positive for meth and heroin.

He insisted nurses give him something to "put out the fire in his head."

One nurse suggested giving the man a water pill and sending him home.

<u>Skin Deep</u>

We've all seen those news stories that make our heads spin. They're the outrageous stories that make you wonder what's wrong with the world. And you think, "That's never going to happen here."

But then it does.

A mentally challenged woman was brought to our ER by way of ambulance. It was a pretty big deal. All available nurses were called to the patient's trauma room, and two doctors were pulled from other cases to respond to the type of emergent situation the department was created to handle.

According to EMS, the patient sustained eight stab wounds to her chest, back, abdomen, breasts, thigh, and temple. As expected, she was hysterical and difficult to treat because she didn't seem to understand the people in her room were there to help, not hurt her more.

"Strangers," she screamed. "I'm not supposed to go with strangers."

Patients in the waiting room moved to the lobby to discuss the shouts that traveled up to the desk. We did our best to move bystanders back to the waiting room.

Our patient was given Ativan and a mental

health duty officer was called in to try to soothe the patient until her mother arrived.

Mom was brought to the hospital by four police officers and was escorted to the patient's room.

According to one of the officers, the patient lived with her mother, father, and aunt. For supper, the patient's mother made spaghetti and garlic bread, the patient's favorite meal. I guess the patient was emotional throughout the evening because her father was unexpectedly required to work overtime.

During the family meal, the patient's mother stepped out of the room and heard the patient's aunt scolding the patient for taking too many meatballs from the pot of spaghetti. The patient's aunt cursed at the woman—the woman with the mental capacity of a child—and ordered her to return the meatballs to the pasta. When the patient attempted to comply, she accidentally dropped her plate on the floor, ruining the meatballs for consumption.

At this point, the aunt grabbed a knife from the table and attacked her niece. The patient's aging mother attempted to stop the attack and sustained a few lacerations to her forearms.

The patient was found to have 13 stab wounds and was listed in critical condition as she was flown out.

Officers arrested the patient's aunt. She's awaiting trial for attempted murder.

YOU SHALL NOT PASS...

...if you come in at 11 p.m., stating you're here to visit Justin Bieber.

I once heard a PA trying to explain to a young mother why it wasn't okay that she filled a bottle with Mountain Dew and gave it to her four-month-old son.

Patient: "You need to tell that doctor I can't take the generic; I'm allergic. He needs to give me a prescription for the real thing."

Me: "So, Dr. So-and-So: this patient doesn't want a generic medication."

Me to Patient: "The doctor said he wrote you that prescription because the brand-name medication is four-hundred-dollars a month and with the insurance you told him about, you can get it for five dollars at Wal Mart."

Patient: "Oh. Never mind, then. I can take this."

Ah, the ER: It's one of the only places you can say, "I hope I don't see you again," and it's taken as a form of endearment.

"How do I know that you would trust me that it was that high if I gave her Tylenol to bring it down?"—a patient's mother, on why she didn't give her child medicine to bring down a 104.6 fever.

You can tell there is a big problem with our society when a dad brings his two-year-old in for drug testing because he heard a rumor that the baby's mother was teaching her how to smoke from a crack pipe.

The baby tested positive.

Titanium

It had been one heck of a long weekend. The first of three nights was one filled with cops bringing in drunk drivers, runners, and violent offenders.

On the second night of the weekend, everything decided to break. Half of my reports were delayed by three hours because the copiers went down in the front and back. In addition to that wonderful news, both scanners up front went out, and I then had no means to copy insurance information. And then my computer software crashed. We were stuck doing everything by hand. Yay for downtime.

The third night wasn't so hectic, but it was steady. But the real action didn't start until 10 minutes before my shift was due to end, when five patients brand new to the hospital arrived one after the other and two code blues/99s were brought in via ambulance.

I prayed in silence over and over, asking for strength and calmness or, maybe even better, that my coworker who just called and said he'd be an hour late…maybe, possibly, miraculously…wouldn't be late after all.

As if we all weren't already having the time of our lives between respiratory and lab running between the two code rooms for stat tests and nurses criss-crossing in the halls to pull patients from the waiting room and try to explain to the coding patients' families that we were in the same boat—waiting for information—well, then something *unique* decided to present.

"Help me," a man groaned as he waddled through the doors. He dropped to his knees and tried crawling to the desk as the families of the codes looked on in shock and confusion.

I hurried to get the man a wheelchair and ask, "What's going on right now?"

"I need help now," he screamed at me, calling me a few curse words in the process.

"Tell me," I ordered slowly, "why you're here today."

"Because I need to see a [f word + ing] doctor. Why else would I be here? Are you retarded?"

One of the family members from one of the coding patients stepped forward. It was only then that I recognized him as one of the deputies on the local police force.

"I suggest you calm yourself down," he told the screaming man, "and if you can't stop battering this girl, I'm going to make sure you find yourself in jail for public disturbance."

The cop started to walk away just as the wife of the wheelchair man started to enter the hospital.

She tossed her hands up in the air and yelled angrily, "Why have you not been taken back yet? What's the purpose of an *emergency room* if they don't treat patients right away?"

"Can you tell me why he's here today?" I asked her.

"Because he needs to see a doctor."

I couldn't help but to look at the ceiling and laugh. Wow.

"Why does he need to see a doctor?" I questioned. "I need a symptom or something in order to sign him in."

"I have something stuck on my dick," he blurted out. There was no way to edit this without capturing the chaos.

Ooooo-kay.

"Now take him to the back," his wife demanded.

"I still need you to come up here and answer a few questions."

"Take me to a doctor NOW," hollered the man.

I looked down and before I closed my eyes to ask for forgiveness for the temper I was about to lose, I could only think, '*My socks are blue? I could have sworn I put on purple socks when I was getting ready.*'

"Why are you just standing there?" screamed the man's wife.

The cop from the waiting room stepped forward again but I waved my hand to hold him off.

"At least two patients are back there *dying* right now," I said sternly. "They're dying. And I have a waiting room full of their families crying and watching you scream because our nurses are too busy shocking someone's heart back to life to come and move you to the back."

I took a breath and continued to the wide-eyed man and his wife, "I understand you're panicking, and you may have a serious problem right now, but please work with me so I can tell someone that you're out here. The more information you can give me, the better. It's very possible another nurse will come and take you before the other patients in the waiting room—all of which who've probably also been wondering why it's taking so long to get to the back."

This man started crying…full-blown bawling.

"I don't want to lose it," he sobbed. "I'm so scared right now."

I nodded and touched the patient's hand. "We'll get you in the system if you or your wife can tell me your name, date of birth, and primary doctor."

The man and his wife took turns giving me the information.

And then the man added, "It hurt on the way here, but now I can't feel it. That's a good sign, right? That means it's easing up?"

With that note, I told the man and his wife to stay at the desk, and I power-walked to find any available nurse.

"Hey," I said, when I found one who was on the way to the front for one of the already-waiting patients. "I need you."

She sighed. "Chest pain?"

I shook my head and smirked. "Not even close."

She raised her brows.

"A man said he has something stuck to his penis and he can't feel it anymore, so I thought I should probably let you guys know so you can check him out."

"He can't feel it at all?"

"That's what he said. He thinks it's a good sign."

"Oh dear."

"Yeah."

The nurse shook her head. "Can you move him on the Tracking Board to three?"

Three was a trauma room. I guess she was going to place him there based on the numbness he felt.

I did as the nurse said as she took the still-crying patient and his now-crying wife to the back.

The cop came up to the desk and gave an upward nod. "What's that all about?"

"HIPAA," I reminded him.

He nodded. "I remember the first time I met that guy. They called me in here because he and his first wife decided they wanted to try to get high by something they saw on the internet."

I was confused.

"The guy put cocaine up his—."

"What?" I cut him off.

"He said he read it gets you high faster than snorting it. I don't even know. But he still had some on him, so he took a little trip to my office that night. Long, long time ago, though. I doubt he even remembers who I am."

The phone rang and I answered.

"Call housekeeping, maintenance, and the fire department," ordered a nurse in a rush. "Ask them if they have anything that can cut through titanium."

"Uh…okay."

"If they do, tell them to get the cutters here now. Like, as in yesterday."

I made the calls, but nobody had cutters with the capability of cutting through titanium. When I relayed this to the nurse, she cursed a whole lot.

I took paperwork to the back and saw now that some of the nurses from the code rooms were in three.

"What in the world is going on?" I asked a unit clerk.

"I guess he and his wife were messing around. They wanted to try one of those ring things, but the only thing they had was his wedding ring."

"No way."

"Way. And now it's stuck."

A nurse from three's room called to the unit clerk to arrange a helicopter pickup from us to a hospital a few hours away.

In the meantime, the nurses tried just about everything they could to get the man's wedding ring off of his appendage. They even huddled around one of the nurses as he YouTubed and Googled solutions to remove stuck rings. Nothing worked, though.

The patient's penis, according to nurses, was turning necrotic upon arrival, and there was no telling how much longer the patient had until he lost his penis to amputation.

In the end, the man was flown out. Unfortunately, we heard the man did lose his penis to the mishap.

And then he went to jail because he ratted himself out after coming off of anesthesia—by detailing how he and his wife were growing marijuana plants and asking his surgeon if she'd be interested in taking some of his pot plants in exchange of slashing his medical bills.

Good Times

I pulled in the parking lot and had no choice but to take the only open space I saw: one located at the very back of the parking lot, at what felt to be a thousand miles away from the ER entrance.

As I was parking, I saw a doctor running through the lot.

"Are you okay?" I asked him, as he neared.

And then I looked toward the entrance and realized the cars parked in the circular drive weren't patients' cars; they were cop cars. Seven cop cars.

I started wondering if the doctor was running because we had a code for an active shooter, thought maybe he could have been running because he desperately needed something from his car, or maybe he had an emergency of his own.

He stopped at the car parked next to mine and said, "It's been a long shift. I'm dying to go home."

I laughed and walked as slowly as I could through the lot, praying all of the police officers would leave before I made it to the door.

They didn't, of course, so I sighed and asked the two evening shift clerks, "What happened now? Is this a drug thing or an MVA?"

One of my coworkers started laughing nervously and shook her head. She was overwhelmed.

"Oh, great," I said, with another sigh. "What is it?"

"Multiple things," said the other clerk. "Two of them are here together…well, kind of. And then they have the others here for three more rooms."

"Yeah," explained the other clerk, trying to keep a straight face. "The two here together are something else."

"What happened?"

Those two, explained my coworkers, taking turns telling the story, were a stepdaughter/stepmother pair. When the teenage daughter fought with the stepmother regarding how she felt it to be unfair that the stepmother's daughter never had to do dishes and never had the same curfew the teenager had, the stepmother grabbed a knife and stabbed the girl. In retaliation, the girl pushed the stepmother…out of a third-story window. The mother didn't die, but she was found to have a broken arm. She was taken to jail.

"And then what else?" I asked.

"Someone drank Pine Sol."

W.T.F… (The periods are in there for a reason—I was thinking this in a slow, drawn-out confusion.)

"I guess they said he didn't drink enough to kill himself. They had to call the poison line and he went upstairs to be admitted."

"Wow."

Both of my coworkers nodded and one said, "And then the guy in room four tried to kill one of the security guards, so now the patient is on the mental health floor, and the security guard is in ICU."

"What?" I exclaimed. "What has been going on here tonight?"

"Another room was just here because the patient was assaulted. Pretty cut and dry thing, really. The girl punched another girl and then got hit back."

Luckily, after my coworkers left, the shift was a calm one.

The patient involved in the strangulation was taken to jail the next morning, while our stepmother was taken to jail as soon as her ER visit was over.

Our mental health patient, somehow, managed to gain access to the housekeeping cart and swiped a bottle of bathroom cleaner. He didn't die after drinking that cleaner, either, but he was transferred out to a facility more equipped to deal with the patient's needs.

<u>Whirrrrrr</u>

This is probably going to be the closest I've been in any of my books of not masking details, and I'm hoping that there are so many videos floating around online that nobody can tell the difference in the video detailed in the story versus all the one out there.

My coworker and I were catching up on the stack of paperwork from the rush of patients who avoided appointments around the holidays, then hurried in to complete the exams and blood tests and all that other not-so-fun-right-before-Christmas-stuff, when a girl walked in with two towels wrapped around her hand.

Not only was she crying, but her friend was also bawling.

"What happened?" I asked.

Now, for the sake of privacy, I'm going to go ahead and change the appliance here.

"I accidentally pressed the button on my food processor as I was trying to get something unstuck from the blades."

"It's bad," the friend said.

I started to get in my 'of course it's bad…they all say that' mood, when the patient unwrapped the towels and held her hand up for us to see.

Okay. It was bad. It was *really* bad.

My coworker called the back and let the charge nurse know we had a trauma case in the lobby. As she was doing that, I sat the patient in a wheelchair—and at a good time, too, because the girl passed out as soon as her butt hit the canvas.

Two nurses ran out front and wheeled the patient back.

Due to a tragic accident, the girl was transferred out and lost four of her fingers.

Let's fast forward a little bit.

My coworker was scrolling through Facebook on her phone and kept showing me videos ranging in topics. We watched Star Wars parodies, tutorials on nails and makeup, animal autopsies, plastic surgery...

"Ew," she said.

That's kind of like my magic word.

"Show me," I said, without even asking what it was about.

She rolled her chair over and held her phone in her palm. She turned the video back by a few seconds and I watched as someone put a hand in a food processor...and then pressed the power button.

The bowl of the processor filled with blood at the person's delayed retraction of his/her mangled hand.

Then the camera person handed the camera (or phone?) to another person, and that person zoomed out on two girls rushing to wrap the injury in a towel.

My coworker hit me in the arm.

There it is, workplace abuse. I think I should be entitled to a week-long paid vacation to Maui or someplace.

"That's that girl!"

Yeah it was.

"Can you play this from the beginning, like, with the sound turned up?"

She did.

We *Mystery Science 3000*ed the heck out of that video. (A lot of our comments didn't make the book because I try to keep stories about work 'clean.') And before you judge, let me tell you we didn't plan on saying anything sarcastic or bad until we heard the opening line of the video.

"Hey," the friend said. "I dare you to put your hand in there and turn it on."

"Yeah," I commented, "you should definitely do that. Did you go to Harvard? Is that where you met this friend?"

The girl replied, "No! Those blades are sharp."

"Nooooo," my coworker said. "Why would you think that?"

"But what's the worst that could happen?" I asked. "They're probably not that sharp, anyway. I bet they can't cut through bone."

"No," the friend said. "The blades stop when they hit something hard. Trust me; I know what I'm talking about. I used to work at [random fast food restaurant]."

"Like, remember when we made smoothies, and, like, the blades chopped up ice and frozen strawberries?" my coworker joked. "Don't worry, though. The blades are only strong enough to cut up those things."

"I worked at that fast food place," I casually noted to my coworker. "And trust *me*, they didn't have food processors when I was there because everything came frozen on the truck."

"Do you think it will hurt when the blades hit my fingers?" asked the patient. She was giggling.

Her friend said no and then added, "Come on. I've been your friend since midterms. Do you think I'd lie to you? Do it. We're going to be famous."

My coworker laughed. "I've known the guy in the waiting room for thirty minutes. Do you think I could convince him to chop off a toe?"

"Do it," I whispered. "Do it. This is going to be something you'll be telling your friends about for the rest of your life. This could be your new Facebook profile picture. Do it."

I'm sure some of you are pretty disgusted on how we added commentary to this video. (I certainly won't lie and pretend to be a more evolved person than I am. I fully believe some situations call for 'DUH!' reactions.) Maybe some of the other close-to-a-million viewers were cringing. Maybe they were doing what we were doing. I don't know.

What I *do* know, though, is that pressing that button was certainly no accident. The patient's fingers hovered above the blades for almost 20 seconds before she shoved them to the bottom of the processor and turned on the appliance. Although the patient was screaming bloody murder, her friends were laughing…right up till the blood started seeping through the first towel.

Comments on the video included arguments between internet users on the validity of the contents. Quite a few people were fairly adamant that it 'just couldn't' be real. One person noted his own tragedy and said the color of the blood was different, so there was 'no way' that happened in reality.

That video has made it over my social media feed at least four times since that happened, and I can't help but to cringe at what I know to be the outcome. The patient even commented on the video a few times and admits what she did was stupid (her words, not mine), and she regrets listening to her friends. She also went on to say they had been drinking and using drugs, and she's mostly taken the criticism (and injury) the best to be expected.

Don't jump the gun and try to figure out which video it is…three other food processor videos hopped through my news feed, too, and though two of them started the same way, they weren't the patient. And, remember, details about the story have been altered to protect patient privacy. If you happen to go looking for the video and think you find it, just remember: there's a good chance that what happened on the video was real, and it was a life-changer for the person involved.

You'd think I'd be over it by now, but I still can't believe so many patients register at three in the morning and tell me they figured they'd better come in now, 'while everyone's asleep' and we're 'not busy.'

Hey, readers!

If you noticed a spelling/grammatical/formatting error in this book, please feel free to review this book and let me know. You deserve the best product, and I don't always catch my mistakes (despite lots of editing and reviewing).

Thank you for your help, and thanks for reading!